Cancer Diet Cookbook for Newly Diagnosed

100+ Nourishing Recipes and Meal Plans to Support Your Journey to Healing and Wellness

By Dr. Melissa Clark

Copyright © 2023 by Dr. Melissa Clark

Table of Contents

Introduction

This Cancer Diet Cookbook for Newly Diagnosed individual is here to offer you guidance and support as you embark on your journey towards better health. Nutrition plays a vital role in your overall well-being, and making informed choices about the foods you eat can have a significant impact on your treatment outcomes and quality of life.

In this cookbook, we'll explore a range of delicious and nourishing recipes specifically designed to meet the unique dietary needs and challenges faced by those who have recently been diagnosed with cancer. Our goal is to provide you with practical and tasty meal options that can help you maintain your strength, manage treatment side effects, and support your body's natural healing processes.

You'll find recipes that are:

1. Nutrient-dense: Packed with vitamins, minerals, and antioxidants to support your immune system and overall health.
2. Easy to prepare: We understand that you might not always have the energy or time to spend hours in the kitchen, so our recipes are designed to be convenient and straightforward.
3. Tailored to your needs: We'll provide guidance on dietary modifications that may be necessary during cancer treatment, such as managing nausea, increasing protein intake, or dealing with specific dietary restrictions.
4. Delicious: We believe that nutritious food should also be enjoyable, and our recipes aim to make healthy eating a pleasure rather than a chore.
5. Adaptable: Every person's journey with cancer is unique, and your dietary needs and preferences may change over time. Our cookbook offers a variety of recipes to accommodate different tastes and dietary requirements.

Remember, the information provided here is not a substitute for medical advice from your healthcare team. It's essential to work closely with your healthcare professionals to create a personalized nutrition plan that aligns with your specific cancer diagnosis and treatment plan.

This cookbook is meant to be a helpful resource, a source of inspiration, and a reminder that you have the strength and support to face the challenges ahead. With the right nutrition and a positive mindset, you can take steps towards a healthier and brighter future.

We wish you the best of luck on your journey to wellness, and we hope that these recipes will be a valuable tool in your cancer-fighting toolkit. Let's get started on the path to better health, one delicious meal at a time.

Chapter 1: Anti-Inflammatory Starters

Turmeric and Ginger Infused Broth

Cook Time: 1 hour

Serving Size: 4

Ingredients:

- 8 cups of water
- 1 inch piece of fresh turmeric, chopped
- 1 inch piece of fresh ginger, chopped
- 1 onion, roughly chopped
- 2 cloves of garlic, minced
- 1 carrot, roughly chopped
- 1 celery stalk, roughly chopped
- 1 tsp sea salt
- Black pepper to taste

Preparation:

1. In a large pot, bring the water to a boil.
2. Add in the chopped turmeric, ginger, onion, garlic, carrot, celery, sea salt, and black pepper.
3. Reduce heat to a simmer and let the broth cook for 1 hour.
4. Using a fine-mesh strainer, strain the broth into a large bowl.
5. You can discard the cooked vegetables or save them for another use.
6. Serve the broth hot and enjoy its immune-boosting benefits.

Avocado and Spinach Smoothie

Cook Time: 5 minutes

Serving Size: 2

Ingredients:

- 1 ripe avocado, peeled and pitted
- 1 cup fresh spinach leaves
- 1 banana, peeled and chopped
- 1 cup unsweetened almond milk
- 1 tsp honey (optional)
- Juice of 1/2 lemon
- Ice cubes (optional)

Preparation:

1. In a blender, combine the avocado, spinach, banana, almond milk, honey (if using), and lemon juice.
2. Blend until smooth and creamy.
3. If desired, add in a couple of ice cubes and blend again.
4. Pour into glasses and serve immediately.

Quinoa Salad with Fresh Herbs

Cook Time: 15 minutes
Serving Size: 4
Ingredients:

- 1 cup quinoa
- 2 cups water
- 1 cup cherry tomatoes, halved
- 1 small cucumber, diced
- 1/4 cup chopped fresh herbs (such as parsley, basil, and mint)
- 1/4 cup crumbled feta cheese
- Juice of 1/2 lemon
- 2 tbsp olive oil
- Salt and black pepper to taste

Preparation:

1. In a medium pot, bring the quinoa and water to a boil.
2. Reduce heat to low, cover, and simmer for 15 minutes.
3. Fluff the quinoa with a fork and let it cool.
4. In a large bowl, combine the cooled quinoa, cherry tomatoes, cucumber, fresh herbs, and feta cheese.
5. In a small bowl, whisk together the lemon juice, olive oil, salt, and black pepper.
6. Pour the dressing over the quinoa mixture and toss to combine.
7. Serve the quinoa salad chilled or at room temperature.

Roasted Beet and Citrus Salad

Cook Time: 30 minutes
Serving Size: 4
Ingredients:

- 3 medium beets
- 2 oranges
- 1 grapefruit
- 1/4 cup sliced red onion

- 1/4 cup crumbled goat cheese
- 2 tbsp balsamic vinegar
- 2 tbsp olive oil
- Salt and black pepper to taste

Preparation:

1. Preheat your oven to 400°F (200°C).
2. Wash and peel the beets and cut them into 1-inch cubes.
3. Place the chopped beets on a baking sheet and drizzle with 1 tablespoon of olive oil.
4. Roast in the oven for 30 minutes, or until tender.
5. While the beets are roasting, peel and slice the oranges and grapefruit into segments.
6. In a small bowl, whisk together the balsamic vinegar, 1 tablespoon of olive oil, salt, and black pepper.
7. In a large bowl, combine the roasted beets, citrus segments, red onion, and goat cheese.
8. Drizzle the dressing over the salad and toss to combine.
9. Serve the roasted beet and citrus salad immediately.

Creamy Cauliflower Soup

Cook Time: 30 minutes
Serving Size: 4
Ingredients:

- 1 large head of cauliflower, chopped into florets
- 4 cups vegetable broth
- 1 onion, chopped
- 3 cloves of garlic, minced
- 1 tsp dried thyme
- 1 tsp dried rosemary
- 1/2 cup heavy cream
- Salt and black pepper to taste
- Fresh herbs for garnish (optional)

Preparation:

1. In a large pot, combine the cauliflower, vegetable broth, onion, garlic, thyme, and rosemary.
2. Bring to a boil, then reduce heat and let the soup simmer for 20 minutes.

3. Use an immersion blender or transfer the soup to a blender and blend until smooth.
4. Stir in the heavy cream and season with salt and black pepper.
5. Serve the creamy cauliflower soup hot, garnished with fresh herbs if desired.

Berry Blast Chia Pudding

Cook Time: Overnight
Serving Size: 4
Ingredients:

- 1 cup unsweetened almond milk
- 1/4 cup chia seeds
- 1 tbsp honey (optional)
- 1 tsp vanilla extract
- 1 cup mixed berries (such as strawberries, blueberries, and raspberries)
- 1/4 cup sliced almonds or chopped walnuts (optional)

Preparation:

1. In a mixing bowl, combine the almond milk, chia seeds, honey (if using), and vanilla extract.
2. Whisk until well combined.
3. Fold in the mixed berries.
4. Divide the chia pudding into 4 individual serving jars or containers.
5. Cover and refrigerate overnight.
6. When ready to serve, top with sliced almonds or chopped walnuts if desired.

Green Tea Infused Miso Soup

Cook Time: 20 minutes
Serving Size: 2
Ingredients:

- 4 cups water
- 1 green tea bag
- 2 tbsp miso paste
- 1 cup cubed tofu
- 1 cup sliced shiitake mushrooms
- 1 cup chopped bok choy

- 1 green onion, chopped
- 1 tsp sesame oil
- Salt and black pepper to taste

Preparation:

1. In a pot, bring the water to a boil.
2. Remove from heat and add in the green tea bag.
3. Let the tea steep for 5 minutes, then discard the tea bag.
4. In a small bowl, dissolve the miso paste in a little bit of water.
5. Add the miso mixture to the pot of green tea and stir well.
6. Bring the soup to a simmer and add in the tofu, mushrooms, and bok choy.
7. Let the soup cook for 10 minutes, until the vegetables are tender.
8. Stir in the green onion, sesame oil, salt, and black pepper.
9. Serve the green tea infused miso soup hot.

Lentil and Vegetable Stew

Cook Time: 45 minutes
Serving Size: 4
Ingredients:

- 2 tbsp olive oil
- 1 onion, chopped
- 2 cloves of garlic, minced
- 2 carrots, diced
- 2 celery stalks, diced
- 1 cup dried lentils, rinsed and drained
- 4 cups vegetable broth
- 2 cups chopped seasonal vegetables (such as zucchini, bell peppers, and green beans)
- 1 tsp dried thyme
- 1 tsp dried oregano
- Salt and black pepper to taste

Preparation:

1. In a large pot, heat the olive oil over medium heat.
2. Add in the onion, garlic, carrots, and celery and cook until softened, about 5 minutes.
3. Stir in the dried lentils, vegetable broth, chopped seasonal vegetables, thyme, oregano, salt, and black pepper.

4. Bring the stew to a boil, then reduce heat and let it simmer for 30 minutes, stirring occasionally.
5. Serve the lentil and vegetable stew hot, garnished with fresh herbs if desired.

Cucumber and Dill Yogurt Dip

Cook Time: 10 minutes
Serving Size: 4
Ingredients:
- 1 cup plain Greek yogurt
- 1 small cucumber, grated and squeezed to remove excess water
- 2 tbsp chopped fresh dill
- 1 clove of garlic, minced
- 1 tsp lemon juice
- Salt and black pepper to taste

Preparation:
1. In a mixing bowl, combine the Greek yogurt, grated cucumber, dill, garlic, lemon juice, salt, and black pepper.
2. Mix well until all ingredients are well combined.
3. Serve the cucumber and dill yogurt dip chilled with your favorite vegetables or pita bread for dipping.

Roasted Red Pepper Hummus

Cook Time: 30 minutes
Serving Size: 4
Ingredients:
- 1 can (15 oz) chickpeas, rinsed and drained
- 1 roasted red pepper, chopped
- 2 cloves of garlic, minced
- 1/4 cup tahini
- 2 tbsp lemon juice
- 2 tbsp olive oil
- Salt and black pepper to taste

Preparation:
1. Preheat your oven to 400°F (200°C).
2. In a baking dish, roast the red pepper for 20 minutes, until slightly charred.
3. In a food processor, combine the chickpeas, roasted red pepper, garlic, tahini, lemon juice, and olive oil.

4. Blend until smooth and creamy.
5. Season with salt and black pepper to taste.
6. Serve the roasted red pepper hummus with pita chips, crackers, or vegetables for dipping.

Chapter 2: Nutrient-Packed Breakfasts

Overnight Oats with Berries

Cook time: 5 minutes

Serving: 1

Ingredients:

- 1/2 cup oats
- 1/2 cup milk (dairy or non-dairy)
- 1/4 cup Greek yogurt
- 1 tbsp chia seeds
- 1 tbsp honey
- 1/4 cup mixed berries (fresh or frozen)

Preparation:

1. In a mason jar or container, add oats, milk, Greek yogurt, chia seeds, and honey.
2. Stir well to combine all ingredients.
3. Top with mixed berries.
4. Cover and refrigerate overnight.
5. In the morning, give the oats a stir and add more milk if desired.
6. Enjoy your creamy and delicious overnight oats with berries!

Sweet Potato and Kale Breakfast Hash

Cook time: 20 minutes

Serving: 2

Ingredients:

- 1 medium sweet potato, diced
- 1 cup kale, chopped
- 1/2 onion, diced
- 2 cloves garlic, minced
- 2 eggs
- Salt and pepper to taste
- Olive oil for cooking

Preparation:

1. Heat a large skillet over medium heat and add a drizzle of olive oil.
2. Add the sweet potato and cook for 8-10 minutes, until tender.
3. Add onion and garlic, and cook for an additional 2 minutes.
4. Stir in kale and cook until wilted, about 2-3 minutes.

5. Create two wells in the mixture and carefully crack an egg into each well.
6. Cover the skillet and let the eggs cook for about 5 minutes, until the whites are set and the yolks are still runny.
7. Once eggs are cooked, sprinkle with salt and pepper.
8. Serve the sweet potato and kale hash with the eggs on top.

Almond Butter and Banana Toast

Cook time: 5 minutes

Serving: 1

Ingredients:

- 2 slices whole grain bread
- 2 tbsp almond butter
- 1 banana, sliced
- 1 tsp honey (optional)
- Chia seeds (optional)

Preparation:

1. Toast two slices of bread until lightly browned.
2. Spread almond butter evenly on each slice.
3. Top with sliced banana.
4. Drizzle honey and sprinkle chia seeds on top, if desired.
5. Enjoy your quick and satisfying almond butter and banana toast!

Spinach and Mushroom Omelette

Cook time: 10 minutes

Serving: 1

Ingredients:

- 2 eggs
- 1 tsp olive oil
- 1 cup spinach
- 1/2 cup sliced mushrooms
- Salt and pepper to taste
- 2 tbsp shredded cheese (optional)

Preparation:

1. Crack two eggs into a bowl and beat with a fork.
2. Heat olive oil in a non-stick skillet over medium heat.
3. Add spinach and mushrooms to the skillet and sauté for 2-3 minutes, until spinach is wilted and mushrooms are cooked.

4. Pour beaten eggs into the skillet over the vegetables.
5. Let the eggs cook for 2-3 minutes, then gently lift the edges of the omelette and tilt the skillet to allow uncooked egg to flow underneath.
6. Once the eggs are mostly set, sprinkle with cheese (if desired) and fold the omelette in half.
7. Let the omelette cook for an additional 2-3 minutes, until cheese is melted and eggs are fully cooked.
8. Sprinkle with salt and pepper and serve your spinach and mushroom omelette hot.

Greek Yogurt Parfait with Honey and Nuts

Cook time: 5 minutes
Serving: 1
Ingredients:
- 1/2 cup Greek yogurt
- 1 tbsp honey
- 2 tbsp chopped nuts (almonds, walnuts, etc.)
- 1/4 cup mixed berries (fresh or frozen)

Preparation:
1. In a bowl or glass, layer Greek yogurt, honey, chopped nuts, and mixed berries.
2. Repeat layers until all ingredients are used.
3. Enjoy your protein-packed and delicious Greek yogurt parfait!

Tofu Scramble with Spinach and Tomatoes

Cook time: 10 minutes
Serving: 2
Ingredients:
- 1/2 block of firm tofu, crumbled
- 1 cup spinach
- 1/2 cup cherry tomatoes, halved
- 1 clove garlic, minced
- 1 tsp turmeric
- Salt and pepper to taste
- Olive oil for cooking

Preparation:
1. Heat olive oil in a skillet over medium heat.

2. Add crumbled tofu to the skillet and season with turmeric, salt, and pepper.
3. Sauté for 2-3 minutes, until tofu is slightly browned.
4. Add spinach, cherry tomatoes, and minced garlic to the skillet and continue to sauté for an additional 2-3 minutes.
5. Once vegetables are cooked, remove from heat and serve your flavorful tofu scramble.

Chia Seed Breakfast Bowl

Cook time: 10 minutes
Serving: 1
Ingredients:
- 1/2 cup chia seeds
- 1 cup milk (dairy or non-dairy)
- 1/2 tsp vanilla extract
- 1/2 cup chopped fruit (mango, kiwi, berries, etc.)
- 2 tbsp shredded coconut
- 1 tbsp honey

Preparation:
1. In a bowl, mix together chia seeds, milk, and vanilla extract.
2. Cover and refrigerate for at least 10 minutes, or overnight.
3. Top the chia seed mixture with chopped fruit, shredded coconut, and a drizzle of honey.
4. Enjoy your nutrient-dense and delicious chia seed breakfast bowl!

Blueberry and Walnut Pancakes

Cook time: 20 minutes
Serving: 2
Ingredients:
- 1 cup flour
- 1 tbsp baking powder
- 1/4 tsp salt
- 1 egg
- 1 cup milk (dairy or non-dairy)
- 2 tbsp melted butter
- 1/2 cup fresh blueberries
- 1/4 cup chopped walnuts
- Maple syrup for serving

Preparation:
1. In a large bowl, mix together flour, baking powder, and salt.
2. In a separate bowl, beat the egg and then stir in the milk and melted butter.
3. Slowly add the wet mixture to the dry mixture, stirring until just combined.
4. Gently fold in the blueberries and chopped walnuts.
5. Heat a griddle or large skillet over medium heat.
6. Using a ladle, pour the pancake batter onto the hot surface, forming 3-4 inch circles.
7. Cook for 2-3 minutes on each side, until golden brown.
8. Serve the blueberry and walnut pancakes with maple syrup.

Quinoa Porridge with Almonds and Raisins

Cook time: 15 minutes
Serving: 2
Ingredients:
- 1 cup cooked quinoa
- 1 cup milk (dairy or non-dairy)
- 1/4 tsp cinnamon
- 1/4 cup chopped almonds
- 1/4 cup raisins
- 1 tbsp honey

Preparation:
1. In a saucepan, combine cooked quinoa, milk, and cinnamon.
2. Heat over medium heat, stirring occasionally, for about 5 minutes.
3. Remove from heat and mix in chopped almonds and raisins.
4. Drizzle with honey and serve your warm and hearty quinoa porridge.

Salmon and Avocado Breakfast Wrap

Cook time: 10 minutes
Serving: 1
Ingredients:
- 1 whole wheat tortilla
- 1/4 avocado, mashed
- 1/4 cup canned salmon, drained
- 1 tsp lemon juice

- Salt and pepper to taste
- 1/4 cup diced tomatoes
- 2 tbsp diced red onion

Preparation:

1. Lay out the tortilla and spread mashed avocado on top.
2. In a small bowl, mix together canned salmon, lemon juice, and salt and pepper.
3. Spread the salmon mixture over the avocado.
4. Top with diced tomatoes and red onion.
5. Roll up the tortilla, tucking in the sides, to create a wrap.
6. Slice the wrap in half and serve your protein-packed and flavorful breakfast wrap.

Chapter 3: Superfood Soups

Roasted Tomato and Basil Soup

Cook time: 45 minutes

Serving: 4-6

Ingredients:

- 2 lbs of ripe tomatoes
- 1 onion, chopped
- 4 cloves of garlic, minced
- 3 cups of vegetable broth
- 1/4 cup of fresh basil leaves, chopped
- 3 tablespoons of olive oil
- Salt and pepper to taste

Preparation:

1. Preheat your oven to 400 degrees Fahrenheit.
2. Cut the tomatoes into quarters and spread them evenly on a baking sheet.
3. Drizzle 2 tablespoons of olive oil over the tomatoes and season with salt and pepper.
4. Roast the tomatoes in the oven for 30 minutes, until they are soft and starting to caramelize.
5. In a large pot, heat the remaining tablespoon of olive oil over medium heat.
6. Add in the onion and garlic, cooking until they are softened, about 5 minutes.
7. Pour in the vegetable broth and bring it to a boil.
8. Add the roasted tomatoes and their juices to the pot, stirring to combine.
9. Let the soup simmer for 10-12 minutes.
10. Using an immersion blender or a regular blender, puree the soup until smooth.
11. Stir in the chopped basil and let the soup simmer for an additional 5 minutes.
12. Serve hot and enjoy the delicious flavors of the roasted tomatoes and basil.

Butternut Squash and Apple Soup

Cook time: 45 minutes

Serving: 4-6

Ingredients:

- 1 large butternut squash, peeled and cubed
- 2 medium apples, chopped
- 1 onion, chopped
- 4 cloves of garlic, minced
- 4 cups of vegetable broth
- 1 teaspoon of ground cinnamon
- 1/4 teaspoon of ground nutmeg
- 1/2 cup of heavy cream (optional)
- Salt and pepper to taste

Preparation:

1. In a large pot, heat some oil over medium-high heat.
2. Add in the chopped onion and garlic, cooking until they are softened, about 5 minutes.
3. Add in the cubed butternut squash and chopped apples, cooking for an additional 5 minutes.
4. Pour in the vegetable broth and bring it to a boil.
5. Reduce the heat and let the soup simmer for 20-25 minutes, until the squash and apples are soft.
6. Using an immersion blender or regular blender, puree the soup until smooth.
7. Season with cinnamon, nutmeg, salt, and pepper.
8. If desired, stir in the heavy cream for a creamier consistency.
9. Let the soup simmer for an additional 5 minutes.
10. Serve hot and enjoy the comforting flavors of butternut squash and apple.

Turmeric and Lentil Soup

Cook time: 40 minutes

Serving: 4-6

Ingredients:

- 1 cup of dried red lentils
- 1 onion, chopped
- 4 cloves of garlic, minced
- 1 tablespoon of turmeric
- 6 cups of vegetable broth
- 1 can of diced tomatoes

- 1 cup of coconut milk
- Salt and pepper to taste

Preparation:

1. In a large pot, heat some oil over medium-high heat.
2. Add in the chopped onion and garlic, cooking until they are softened, about 5 minutes.
3. Add in the dried lentils and turmeric, cooking for an additional 2 minutes.
4. Pour in the vegetable broth and bring it to a boil.
5. Reduce the heat and let the soup simmer for 20 minutes, until the lentils are soft.
6. Add in the diced tomatoes and coconut milk, stirring to combine.
7. Let the soup simmer for an additional 5 minutes.
8. Season with salt and pepper to taste.
9. Serve hot and enjoy the warm and comforting flavors of turmeric and lentils.

Spinach and Chickpea Soup

Cook time: 30 minutes

Serving: 4-6

Ingredients:

- 1 onion, chopped
- 4 cloves of garlic, minced
- 1 can of chickpeas, drained and rinsed
- 4 cups of vegetable broth
- 1 cup of chopped spinach
- Juice of 1 lemon
- 1 teaspoon of dried oregano
- Salt and pepper to taste

Preparation:

1. In a large pot, heat some oil over medium-high heat.
2. Add in the chopped onion and garlic, cooking until they are softened, about 5 minutes.
3. Add in the drained and rinsed chickpeas, cooking for an additional 3 minutes.
4. Pour in the vegetable broth and bring it to a boil.
5. Reduce the heat and let the soup simmer for 10 minutes.

6. Add in the chopped spinach, lemon juice, and oregano, stirring to combine.
7. Let the soup simmer for an additional 5 minutes.
8. Season with salt and pepper to taste.
9. Serve hot and enjoy the wholesome flavors of spinach and chickpeas.

Carrot and Ginger Soup

Cook time: 30 minutes
Serving: 4-6
Ingredients:
- 1 onion, chopped
- 4 cloves of garlic, minced
- 1 lb of carrots, peeled and chopped
- 1 tablespoon of grated ginger
- 4 cups of vegetable broth
- 1 cup of coconut milk
- Salt and pepper to taste

Preparation:
1. In a large pot, heat some oil over medium-high heat.
2. Add in the chopped onion and garlic, cooking until they are softened, about 5 minutes.
3. Add in the chopped carrots and grated ginger, cooking for an additional 5 minutes.
4. Pour in the vegetable broth and bring it to a boil.
5. Reduce the heat and let the soup simmer for 20 minutes, until the carrots are soft.
6. Using an immersion blender or regular blender, puree the soup until smooth.
7. Stir in the coconut milk and let the soup simmer for an additional 5 minutes.
8. Season with salt and pepper to taste.
9. Serve hot and enjoy the warming flavors of carrots and ginger.

Broccoli and Kale Detox Soup

Cook time: 30 minutes
Serving: 4-6
Ingredients:

- 1 onion, chopped
- 4 cloves of garlic, minced
- 1 head of broccoli, chopped
- 2 cups of chopped kale
- 4 cups of vegetable broth
- 1 cup of almond milk
- 1/4 cup of nutritional yeast
- 1 teaspoon of dried thyme
- Salt and pepper to taste

Preparation:

1. In a large pot, heat some oil over medium-high heat.
2. Add in the chopped onion and garlic, cooking until they are softened, about 5 minutes.
3. Add in the chopped broccoli and kale, cooking for an additional 5 minutes.
4. Pour in the vegetable broth and bring it to a boil.
5. Reduce the heat and let the soup simmer for 15 minutes, until the vegetables are soft.
6. Using an immersion blender or regular blender, puree the soup until smooth.
7. Stir in the almond milk and nutritional yeast, and let the soup simmer for an additional 5 minutes.
8. Season with dried thyme, salt, and pepper to taste.
9. Serve hot and enjoy the detoxifying flavors of broccoli and kale.

Creamy Mushroom and Barley Soup

Cook time: 50 minutes

Serving: 4-6

Ingredients:

- 1 onion, chopped
- 4 cloves of garlic, minced
- 1 lb of mushrooms, thinly sliced
- 1 cup of pearl barley
- 4 cups of vegetable broth
- 1 cup of heavy cream
- 1/4 cup of chopped parsley
- Salt and pepper to taste

Preparation:

1. In a large pot, heat some oil over medium-high heat.
2. Add in the chopped onion and garlic, cooking until they are softened, about 5 minutes.
3. Add in the sliced mushrooms and cook for an additional 5 minutes.
4. Pour in the vegetable broth and bring it to a boil.
5. Add in the pearl barley and let the soup simmer for 30 minutes, until the barley is cooked.
6. Stir in the heavy cream and let the soup simmer for an additional 5 minutes.
7. Season with chopped parsley, salt, and pepper.
8. Serve hot and enjoy the creamy and earthy flavors of mushrooms and barley.

Miso and Seaweed Soup

Cook time: 20 minutes
Serving: 4-6
Ingredients:
- 4 cups of vegetable broth
- 2 cups of water
- 1/4 cup of miso paste
- 1 cup of diced tofu
- 1/2 cup of sliced seaweed
- 1 green onion, sliced

Preparation:
1. In a large pot, bring the vegetable broth and 2 cups of water to a boil.
2. Reduce the heat and let it simmer.
3. Ladle out 1/2 cup of the broth into a small bowl and mix in the miso paste until smooth.
4. Pour the miso mixture back into the pot and stir.
5. Add in the diced tofu and sliced seaweed.
6. Let the soup simmer for 5 minutes.
7. Serve hot and garnish with sliced green onions.

Creamy Cauliflower and Turmeric Soup

Cook time: 30 minutes
Serving: 4-6

Ingredients:

- 1 onion, chopped
- 4 cloves of garlic, minced
- 1 head of cauliflower, chopped
- 4 cups of vegetable broth
- 1 cup of coconut milk
- 1 teaspoon of ground turmeric
- Salt and pepper to taste

Preparation:

1. In a large pot, heat some oil over medium-high heat.
2. Add in the chopped onion and garlic, cooking until they are softened, about 5 minutes.
3. Add in the chopped cauliflower and cook for an additional 5 minutes.
4. Pour in the vegetable broth and bring it to a boil.
5. Reduce the heat and let the soup simmer for 20 minutes, until the cauliflower is soft.
6. Using an immersion blender or regular blender, puree the soup until smooth.
7. Stir in the coconut milk and turmeric, and let the soup simmer for an additional 5 minutes.
8. Season with salt and pepper to taste.
9. Serve hot and enjoy the creamy and flavorful combination of cauliflower and turmeric.

Red Lentil and Spinach Soup

Cook time: 30 minutes

Serving: 4-6

Ingredients:

- 1 onion, chopped
- 4 cloves of garlic, minced
- 1 cup of dried red lentils
- 4 cups of vegetable broth
- 1 can of diced tomatoes
- 2 cups of chopped spinach
- 1 teaspoon of dried basil
- Salt and pepper to taste

Preparation:

1. In a large pot, heat some oil over medium-high heat.
2. Add in the chopped onion and garlic, cooking until they are softened, about 5 minutes.
3. Add in the dried red lentils and cook for an additional 2 minutes.
4. Pour in the vegetable broth and bring it to a boil.
5. Reduce the heat and let the soup simmer for 20 minutes, until the lentils are soft.
6. Add in the diced tomatoes and chopped spinach, stirring to combine.
7. Let the soup simmer for an additional 5 minutes.
8. Season with dried basil, salt, and pepper to taste.
9. Serve hot and enjoy the hearty and nutritious flavors of red lentils and spinach.

Chapter 4: Healthy Salads

Kale and Quinoa Salad with Lemon Vinaigrette

Cook time: 20 minutes

Serving: 4

Ingredients:

- 1 cup quinoa
- 2 cups water
- 1 bunch of kale, stems removed and chopped
- 1 cup cherry tomatoes, halved
- 1 avocado, diced
- 1/4 cup diced red onion
- 1/4 cup crumbled feta cheese
- 1/4 cup chopped fresh herbs (such as cilantro, parsley, or basil)
- Salt and pepper to taste

Lemon Vinaigrette:

- 1/4 cup olive oil
- 2 tablespoons lemon juice
- 1 teaspoon Dijon mustard
- 1 garlic clove, minced
- 1 teaspoon honey
- Salt and pepper to taste

Preparation:

1. In a medium pot, bring water to a boil and add quinoa. Reduce heat to low, cover, and simmer for 15 minutes. Remove from heat and let cool.
2. In a large bowl, add cooled quinoa, kale, tomatoes, avocado, red onion, feta cheese, and herbs.
3. In a small bowl, whisk together olive oil, lemon juice, Dijon mustard, garlic, honey, salt, and pepper to make the vinaigrette.
4. Pour the vinaigrette over the salad and toss to combine.
5. Serve and enjoy!

Watermelon and Feta Salad

Cook time: 15 minutes

Serving: 4

Ingredients:

- 4 cups cubed watermelon

- 1/2 cup crumbled feta cheese
- 1/4 cup thinly sliced red onion
- 1/4 cup chopped fresh mint
- 2 tablespoons balsamic vinegar
- 2 tablespoons extra virgin olive oil
- 1 teaspoon honey
- Salt and pepper to taste

Preparation:

1. In a large bowl, combine watermelon, feta cheese, red onion, and mint.
2. In a small bowl, whisk together balsamic vinegar, olive oil, honey, salt, and pepper to make the dressing.
3. Pour the dressing over the salad and toss to combine.
4. Serve and enjoy!

Beet and Walnut Salad with Goat Cheese

Cook time: 30 minutes

Serving: 4

Ingredients:

- 4 medium beets, peeled and thinly sliced
- 1/2 cup chopped walnuts
- 1/4 cup crumbled goat cheese
- 2 cups mixed greens
- 2 tablespoons extra virgin olive oil
- 1 tablespoon balsamic vinegar
- 1 teaspoon Dijon mustard
- 1 teaspoon honey
- Salt and pepper to taste

Preparation:

1. Preheat oven to 375 degrees F.
2. Place sliced beets on a baking sheet lined with foil. Drizzle with olive oil and sprinkle with salt and pepper.
3. Bake for 25-30 minutes, until beets are tender.
4. In a small bowl, whisk together olive oil, balsamic vinegar, Dijon mustard, honey, salt, and pepper to make the dressing.
5. In a large bowl, combine roasted beets, walnuts, goat cheese, and mixed greens. Pour dressing over the salad and toss to combine.
6. Serve and enjoy!

Avocado and Black Bean Salad

Cook time: 15 minutes

Serving: 4

Ingredients:

- 1 can black beans, drained and rinsed
- 2 avocados, diced
- 1 cup cherry tomatoes, halved
- 1/4 cup diced red onion
- 1/4 cup chopped cilantro
- Juice of 1 lime
- 2 tablespoons extra virgin olive oil
- 1 teaspoon cumin
- Salt and pepper to taste

Preparation:

1. In a medium bowl, combine black beans, avocados, cherry tomatoes, red onion, and cilantro.
2. In a small bowl, whisk together lime juice, olive oil, cumin, salt, and pepper to make the dressing.
3. Pour the dressing over the salad and toss to combine.
4. Serve and enjoy!

Spinach and Strawberry Salad

Cook time: 15 minutes

Serving: 4

Ingredients:

- 4 cups baby spinach
- 1 cup sliced strawberries
- 1/4 cup crumbled feta cheese
- 1/4 cup chopped almonds
- 2 tablespoons balsamic vinegar
- 2 tablespoons extra virgin olive oil
- 1 teaspoon Dijon mustard
- 1 teaspoon honey
- Salt and pepper to taste

Preparation:

1. In a large bowl, combine baby spinach, sliced strawberries, feta cheese, and almonds.

2. In a small bowl, whisk together balsamic vinegar, olive oil, Dijon mustard, honey, salt, and pepper to make the dressing.
3. Pour the dressing over the salad and toss to combine.
4. Serve and enjoy!

Mediterranean Chickpea Salad

Cook time: 15 minutes
Serving: 4
Ingredients:
- 2 cups canned chickpeas, drained and rinsed
- 1 cup diced cucumber
- 1 cup diced tomatoes
- 1/2 cup diced red onion
- 1/4 cup chopped Kalamata olives
- 1/4 cup crumbled feta cheese
- 2 tablespoons extra virgin olive oil
- Juice of 1 lemon
- 1 clove garlic, minced
- 1 teaspoon dried oregano
- Salt and pepper to taste

Preparation:
1. In a large bowl, combine chickpeas, cucumber, tomatoes, red onion, olives, and feta cheese.
2. In a small bowl, whisk together olive oil, lemon juice, garlic, oregano, salt, and pepper to make the dressing.
3. Pour the dressing over the salad and toss to combine.
4. Serve and enjoy!

Cabbage and Apple Slaw

Cook time: 15 minutes
Serving: 4
Ingredients:
- 2 cups shredded green cabbage
- 1 cup shredded red cabbage
- 1 cup grated carrots
- 1 apple, diced
- 1/4 cup chopped almonds
- 2 tablespoons apple cider vinegar

- 2 tablespoons extra virgin olive oil
- 1 teaspoon Dijon mustard
- 1 teaspoon honey
- Salt and pepper to taste

Preparation:

1. In a large bowl, combine green cabbage, red cabbage, carrots, apple, and almonds.
2. In a small bowl, whisk together apple cider vinegar, olive oil, Dijon mustard, honey, salt, and pepper to make the dressing.
3. Pour the dressing over the slaw and toss to combine.
4. Serve and enjoy!

Thai-Inspired Peanut Salad

Cook time: 15 minutes
Serving: 4
Ingredients:

- 4 cups mixed greens
- 1 cup sliced cucumber
- 1 cup shredded carrots
- 1/2 cup thinly sliced red onion
- 1/4 cup chopped cilantro
- 1/4 cup chopped peanuts
- 2 tablespoons soy sauce
- 2 tablespoons rice vinegar
- 2 tablespoons sesame oil
- 1 tablespoon honey
- 1 clove garlic, minced
- 1 teaspoon grated ginger

Preparation:

1. In a large bowl, combine mixed greens, cucumber, carrots, red onion, and cilantro.
2. In a small bowl, whisk together soy sauce, rice vinegar, sesame oil, honey, garlic, and ginger to make the dressing.
3. Pour the dressing over the salad and toss to combine.
4. Sprinkle chopped peanuts on top and serve.

Roasted Vegetable and Couscous Salad

Cook time: 30 minutes

Serving: 4
Ingredients:
- 1 cup couscous
- 1 cup water
- 1 red bell pepper, sliced
- 1 yellow bell pepper, sliced
- 1 zucchini, sliced
- 1 red onion, sliced
- 1 cup cherry tomatoes, halved
- 1/4 cup crumbled feta cheese
- 2 tablespoons balsamic vinegar
- 2 tablespoons extra virgin olive oil
- 1 teaspoon Dijon mustard
- 1 teaspoon honey
- Salt and pepper to taste

Preparation:
1. Preheat oven to 375 degrees F.
2. In a large bowl, add couscous and water. Let sit for 10 minutes, then fluff with a fork.
3. On a baking sheet lined with foil, place sliced bell peppers, zucchini, and red onion. Drizzle with olive oil and sprinkle with salt and pepper. Roast for 25 minutes, until vegetables are tender.
4. In a small bowl, whisk together balsamic vinegar, olive oil, Dijon mustard, honey, salt, and pepper to make the dressing.
5. In a large bowl, combine cooked couscous, roasted vegetables, cherry tomatoes, and feta cheese. Pour dressing over the salad and toss to combine.
6. Serve and enjoy!

Arugula and Pear Salad with Balsamic Dressing

Cook time: 15 minutes
Serving: 4
Ingredients:
- 4 cups arugula
- 1 pear, sliced
- 1/4 cup crumbled goat cheese
- 1/4 cup chopped walnuts
- 2 tablespoons balsamic vinegar

- 2 tablespoons extra virgin olive oil
- 1 teaspoon Dijon mustard
- 1 teaspoon honey
- Salt and pepper to taste

Preparation:

1. In a large bowl, combine arugula, sliced pear, goat cheese, and walnuts.
2. In a small bowl, whisk together balsamic vinegar, olive oil, Dijon mustard, honey, salt, and pepper to make the dressing.
3. Pour the dressing over the salad and toss to combine.
4. Serve and enjoy!

Chapter 5: Lean Protein Dishes

Grilled Chicken with Lemon and Herbs

Cook time: 20 minutes

Serving: 4

Ingredients:

- 4 boneless, skinless chicken breasts
- 1/4 cup olive oil
- juice of 1 lemon
- 2 cloves of garlic, minced
- 1 tsp dried oregano
- 1 tsp dried thyme
- 1 tsp dried rosemary
- salt and pepper to taste

Preparation:

1. In a small bowl, whisk together olive oil, lemon juice, minced garlic, oregano, thyme, rosemary, salt and pepper.
2. Place chicken breasts in a large resealable bag and pour marinade over them. Seal the bag and gently massage the marinade into the chicken. Let it marinate in the refrigerator for at least 30 minutes or up to 4 hours.
3. Preheat grill to medium-high heat. Remove chicken from marinade and discard remaining marinade.
4. Grill chicken for about 8-10 minutes per side, or until the internal temperature reaches 165°F (74°C).
5. Let the chicken rest for 5 minutes before serving.

Baked Salmon with Dill and Asparagus

Cook time: 20 minutes

Serving: 4

Ingredients:

- 4 salmon fillets
- 1 bunch asparagus, trimmed
- 1 tbsp olive oil
- 2 cloves of garlic, minced
- 1 tsp dried dill
- salt and pepper to taste
- lemon wedges for serving

Preparation:
1. Preheat oven to 400°F (200°C) and line a baking sheet with parchment paper.
2. Place salmon fillets on the parchment paper and season with salt and pepper.
3. In a small bowl, mix together olive oil, minced garlic, and dried dill. Drizzle over the salmon fillets.
4. Place asparagus on the baking sheet beside the salmon. Drizzle with olive oil and season with salt and pepper.
5. Bake for 15-20 minutes, or until the salmon is cooked through and the asparagus is tender.
6. Serve with lemon wedges.

Quinoa and Black Bean Stuffed Peppers

Cook time: 30 minutes

Serving: 6

Ingredients:
- 6 bell peppers (any color)
- 1 cup quinoa, rinsed and drained
- 1 tbsp olive oil
- 1 onion, diced
- 2 cloves of garlic, minced
- 1 can black beans, rinsed and drained
- 1 can diced tomatoes
- 1 cup corn kernels (fresh or frozen)
- 1 tsp chili powder
- 1 tsp cumin
- salt and pepper to taste
- 1 cup shredded cheddar cheese (optional)
- fresh cilantro for serving (optional)

Preparation:
1. Preheat oven to 375°F (190°C). Cut the tops off the bell peppers and remove the seeds and membranes. Place them in a baking dish and set aside.
2. In a saucepan, bring 2 cups of water to a boil. Add in the quinoa, reduce heat, and let it simmer for 15 minutes.
3. In a skillet, heat olive oil over medium heat. Add in onion and garlic and cook until softened. Then add in black beans, diced

tomatoes, corn, chili powder, and cumin. Stir and let it cook for another 5-7 minutes.
4. Once the quinoa is cooked, add it to the skillet with the bean and vegetable mixture. Stir to combine. Season with salt and pepper.
5. Scoop the quinoa mixture into the bell peppers, filling them to the top. If desired, top with shredded cheese.
6. Bake for 20 minutes, or until peppers are tender and filling is heated through.
7. Serve with fresh cilantro, if desired.

Tofu Stir-Fry with Broccoli and Cashews

Cook time: 20 minutes

Serving: 4

Ingredients:

- 12 oz block of firm tofu
- 2 tbsp cornstarch
- 3 tbsp soy sauce
- 2 cloves of garlic, minced
- 1 tbsp grated ginger
- 1 tbsp sesame oil
- 1 tbsp olive oil
- 3 cups broccoli florets
- 1 cup cashews
- cooked brown rice for serving

Preparation:

1. Cut tofu into 1-inch cubes and place them in a bowl. Sprinkle cornstarch over the tofu and toss to coat evenly.
2. In a small bowl, mix together soy sauce, minced garlic, grated ginger, and sesame oil. Set aside.
3. In a large skillet, heat olive oil over medium-high heat. Add in tofu and cook until golden brown, about 5 minutes per side.
4. Remove tofu from skillet and set aside.
5. In the same skillet, add in broccoli and stir-fry for 3-5 minutes until tender.
6. Add the tofu back to the skillet and pour the soy sauce mixture over the tofu and broccoli. Stir to combine and cook for another 2-3 minutes.
7. Serve with cooked brown rice and top with cashews.

Lentil and Vegetable Curry

Cook time: 45 minutes

Serving: 6

Ingredients:

- 1 cup dried lentils, rinsed and drained
- 2 tbsp olive oil
- 1 onion, diced
- 2 cloves of garlic, minced
- 1 tbsp grated ginger
- 1 bell pepper, diced
- 1 zucchini, diced
- 1 cup cauliflower florets
- 1 can diced tomatoes
- 1 can coconut milk
- 1 tbsp curry powder
- 1 tsp cumin
- 1 tsp turmeric
- salt and pepper to taste
- fresh cilantro for serving (optional)

Preparation:

1. In a saucepan, bring 2 cups of water to a boil. Add in the lentils, reduce heat, and let it simmer for 20 minutes.
2. In a large pot, heat olive oil over medium heat. Add in onion, garlic, and ginger and cook until softened.
3. Add in bell pepper, zucchini, and cauliflower to the pot. Cook for 5 minutes.
4. Once lentils are cooked, add them to the pot with the vegetables.
5. Pour in diced tomatoes and coconut milk. Stir to combine.
6. Add in curry powder, cumin, turmeric, salt and pepper. Stir and let it simmer for another 10-15 minutes.
7. Serve over rice and top with fresh cilantro, if desired.

Turkey and Spinach Meatballs

Cook time: 25 minutes

Serving: 4

Ingredients:

- 1 lb ground turkey

- 1 cup spinach, chopped
- 1/2 cup breadcrumbs
- 1 egg
- 2 cloves of garlic, minced
- 1 tbsp grated parmesan cheese
- 1 tsp dried oregano
- salt and pepper to taste

Preparation:

1. Preheat oven to 375°F (190°C) and line a baking sheet with parchment paper.
2. In a large bowl, combine ground turkey, chopped spinach, breadcrumbs, egg, minced garlic, grated parmesan cheese, oregano, salt and pepper.
3. Mix well using your hands and then shape the mixture into small balls.
4. Place meatballs on the prepared baking sheet and bake for 20-25 minutes, or until cooked through.
5. Serve with your choice of pasta and marinara sauce.

Seared Tuna with Sesame Seeds

Cook time: 10 minutes

Serving: 2

Ingredients:

- 2 tuna steaks
- salt and pepper to taste
- 2 tbsp soy sauce
- 2 tsp honey
- 2 tsp rice vinegar
- 1 tbsp sesame oil
- 2 tbsp sesame seeds
- 1 tbsp olive oil
- 1 green onion, chopped for garnish (optional)

Preparation:

1. Season tuna steaks with salt and pepper.
2. In a small bowl, mix together soy sauce, honey, rice vinegar, and sesame oil.
3. Coat the tuna steaks with sesame seeds on both sides, pressing gently to ensure they stick.

4. Heat olive oil in a skillet over high heat. Once hot, add in the tuna steaks and cook for 1-2 minutes per side, depending on desired level of doneness.
5. Pour the soy sauce mixture into the skillet and toss the tuna steaks for 30 seconds.
6. Serve immediately and garnish with chopped green onions, if desired.

Grilled Shrimp and Mango Salsa

Cook time: 15 minutes
Serving: 4
Ingredients:
For the Shrimp:

- 1 lb raw shrimp, peeled and deveined
- 1 tbsp olive oil
- 1 tsp chili powder
- 1 tsp garlic powder
- salt and pepper to taste

For the Mango Salsa:

- 1 mango, diced
- 1/4 cup red onion, diced
- 1 jalapeno, seeded and minced
- juice of 1 lime
- 1 tbsp chopped cilantro (optional)

Preparation:

1. In a small bowl, mix together olive oil, chili powder, garlic powder, salt and pepper. Coat the shrimp in this mixture.
2. Heat a grill or grill pan to medium-high heat. Grill shrimp for 2-3 minutes per side, or until cooked through.
3. In another small bowl, mix together diced mango, red onion, jalapeno, lime juice, and cilantro.
4. Serve grilled shrimp with mango salsa on top.

Lemon Garlic Baked Cod

Cook time: 20 minutes
Serving: 4
Ingredients:

- 4 cod fillets

- 1/4 cup butter, melted
- 2 cloves of garlic, minced
- juice of 1 lemon
- 1 tsp dried parsley
- salt and pepper to taste
- lemon wedges for serving

Preparation:

1. Preheat oven to 375°F (190°C) and line a baking dish with parchment paper.
2. Place cod fillets in the prepared baking dish.
3. In a small bowl, mix together melted butter, minced garlic, lemon juice, dried parsley, salt and pepper.
4. Pour the mixture over the cod fillets, making sure they are evenly coated.
5. Bake for 15-20 minutes, or until the fish is cooked through and flakes easily with a fork.
6. Serve with lemon wedges.

Tempeh and Vegetable Skewers

Cook time: 15 minutes

Serving: 4

Ingredients:

- 8 oz tempeh, cut into cubes
- 1 bell pepper, diced
- 1 zucchini, cut into rounds
- 8 cherry tomatoes
- 1/4 cup olive oil
- 2 cloves of garlic, minced
- 1 tsp dried oregano
- 1 tsp dried basil
- salt and pepper to taste

Preparation:

1. Preheat grill to medium-high heat.
2. On skewers, alternate tempeh, bell pepper, zucchini, and cherry tomatoes.
3. In a small bowl, mix together olive oil, minced garlic, oregano, basil, salt and pepper.
4. Brush the skewers with the olive oil mixture.

5. Grill for 5-7 minutes per side, or until vegetables are tender.
6. Serve immediately.

Chapter 6: Plant-Based Delights

Eggplant and Chickpea Tagine

Cook time: 45 minutes

Serving: 4-6 servings

Ingredients:

- 1 large eggplant, cut into 1-inch cubes
- 1 onion, finely chopped
- 3 garlic cloves, minced
- 1 can (15 oz) chickpeas, drained and rinsed
- 1 can (14.5 oz) diced tomatoes
- 1/4 cup vegetable broth
- 1 tsp ground cumin
- 1 tsp ground coriander
- 1 tsp paprika
- 1/4 tsp cinnamon
- Salt and pepper, to taste
- Fresh parsley or cilantro, for garnish
- Cooked couscous or rice, for serving

Preparation:

1. In a large pot or Dutch oven, heat 1 tbsp of oil over medium heat. Add the eggplant cubes and cook until golden brown, about 5-7 minutes. Remove the eggplant from the pot and set aside.
2. In the same pot, add the onion and garlic and cook until softened, about 3 minutes.
3. Add the drained chickpeas, diced tomatoes, vegetable broth, cumin, coriander, paprika, cinnamon, salt and pepper to the pot. Stir to combine.
4. Return the eggplant to the pot and bring the mixture to a boil. Reduce the heat to low and let simmer for 20-25 minutes, stirring occasionally.
5. Serve over cooked couscous or rice, and garnish with fresh parsley or cilantro. Enjoy!

Vegan Lentil Shepherd's Pie

Cook time: 1 hour

Serving: 6-8 servings

Ingredients:

- 2 cups green lentils, rinsed and drained
- 4 cups water or vegetable broth
- 1 onion, finely chopped
- 3 carrots, peeled and chopped
- 3 stalks celery, chopped
- 2 garlic cloves, minced
- 1 cup frozen peas
- 1 tbsp tomato paste
- 2 tbsp soy sauce
- 1 tsp dried thyme
- 1 tsp dried rosemary
- Salt and pepper, to taste
- 4 cups mashed potatoes (use vegan butter/milk if desired)

Preparation:

1. In a large pot, combine the lentils and water or vegetable broth. Bring to a boil, then reduce the heat and let simmer for 15-20 minutes, until the lentils are tender.
2. Preheat your oven to 375°F (190°C).
3. In a separate pan, heat 1 tbsp oil over medium heat. Add the onion and cook until softened, about 3 minutes. Then add the chopped carrots, celery, and garlic, and cook for an additional 5 minutes.
4. Add the frozen peas, tomato paste, soy sauce, dried thyme, dried rosemary, salt and pepper to the pan. Stir to combine, and cook for a few more minutes until the vegetables are tender.
5. In a 9x13 inch baking dish, spread the cooked lentils evenly. Top with the vegetable mixture, spreading it evenly. Top with mashed potatoes, spreading them evenly over the vegetables.
6. Bake for 30 minutes, until the potatoes are golden brown. Let cool for a few minutes before serving. Enjoy!

Portobello Mushroom Burgers

Cook time: 30 minutes

Serving: 4 burgers

Ingredients:

- 4 large portobello mushroom caps, cleaned and stems removed
- 2 tbsp balsamic vinegar
- 2 tbsp olive oil

- 2 garlic cloves, minced
- 1 tsp dried thyme
- Salt and pepper, to taste
- 4 burger buns
- Toppings of your choice (lettuce, onion, tomato)

Preparation:

1. In a small bowl, mix together the balsamic vinegar, olive oil, minced garlic, dried thyme, salt and pepper.
2. Place the cleaned mushroom caps in a pan or dish and pour the marinade over them, making sure to coat both sides. Let marinate for 15 minutes.
3. Preheat a grill or grill pan over medium heat, and lightly oil the surface.
4. Place the marinated mushroom caps on the grill and cook for 5-7 minutes on each side, until tender and slightly charred.
5. Serve on a bun with your desired toppings. Enjoy!

Zucchini Noodles with Pesto

Cook time: 15 minutes

Serving: 2 servings

Ingredients:

- 2 large zucchinis
- 1/4 cup basil pesto
- 1 tbsp olive oil
- 2 garlic cloves, minced
- 1/4 cup cherry tomatoes, halved
- Salt and pepper, to taste
- Crushed red pepper flakes (optional)

Preparation:

1. Using a spiralizer, turn the zucchinis into noodles.
2. In a large pan, heat the olive oil over medium heat. Add the minced garlic and cook for 1-2 minutes, until fragrant.
3. Add the zucchini noodles to the pan and cook for 3-4 minutes, until they start to soften.
4. Add the basil pesto to the pan and stir to combine with the zucchini noodles. Cook for an additional 2-3 minutes.
5. Add the halved cherry tomatoes and season with salt and pepper (and crushed red pepper flakes if desired).

6. Serve hot and enjoy!

Stuffed Bell Peppers with Quinoa and Black Beans

Cook time: 45 minutes
Serving: 4 servings
Ingredients:

- 4 bell peppers, halved and seeded
- 1 cup quinoa, rinsed and drained
- 1 can (15 oz) black beans, drained and rinsed
- 1 onion, finely chopped
- 3 garlic cloves, minced
- 1 can (14.5 oz) diced tomatoes
- 1 cup vegetable broth
- 1 tsp ground cumin
- 1 tsp chili powder
- Salt and pepper, to taste
- 1/2 cup shredded vegan cheese (optional)
- Fresh cilantro, for garnish

Preparation:

1. Preheat your oven to 375°F (190°C).
2. In a large pot, bring 2 cups of water to a boil. Add the quinoa, reduce the heat and let simmer for 15 minutes, until cooked and fluffy.
3. In a large skillet, heat 1 tbsp oil over medium heat. Add the chopped onion and garlic and cook for 3-5 minutes, until soft.
4. Add the cooked quinoa, black beans, diced tomatoes, vegetable broth, ground cumin, chili powder, salt and pepper to the skillet. Stir to combine and let cook for a few more minutes.
5. Arrange the halved bell peppers in a 9x13 inch baking dish. Spoon the quinoa and black bean mixture into each pepper half.
6. If using, top with shredded vegan cheese.
7. Bake for 25 minutes, until the peppers are tender and the cheese is melted. Garnish with fresh cilantro before serving. Enjoy!

Vegan Pad Thai with Tofu

Cook time: 25 minutes

Serving: 4 servings

Ingredients:

- 8 oz rice noodles
- 1 tbsp vegetable oil
- 1 block (14 oz) extra firm tofu, drained and diced
- 1 onion, finely chopped
- 2 garlic cloves, minced
- 1 red bell pepper, thinly sliced
- 1 cup shredded carrot
- 1 cup bean sprouts
- 1/4 cup chopped peanuts
- Fresh cilantro, for garnish

Sauce ingredients:

- 1/4 cup soy sauce
- 3 tbsp maple syrup
- 2 tbsp lime juice
- 2 tbsp rice vinegar
- 1 tbsp chili garlic sauce
- 1 tsp sesame oil

Preparation:

1. Cook the rice noodles according to package instructions. Drain and set aside.
2. In a small bowl, mix together the sauce ingredients.
3. In a large skillet or wok, heat the vegetable oil over medium heat. Add the diced tofu and cook until golden brown, about 5 minutes.
4. Add the chopped onion, minced garlic, and red bell pepper to the skillet. Cook for 3-5 minutes, until the vegetables start to soften.
5. Add the cooked rice noodles and sauce to the skillet. Stir to combine and let cook for a few more minutes.
6. Add the shredded carrot and bean sprouts to the skillet, and cook for an additional 2-3 minutes.
7. Serve hot, topped with chopped peanuts and fresh cilantro. Enjoy!

Sweet Potato and Black Bean Enchiladas

Cook time: 45 minutes

Serving: 6 servings

Ingredients:

- 2 large sweet potatoes, peeled and diced
- 2 tbsp olive oil
- 1 onion, finely chopped
- 2 garlic cloves, minced
- 1 can (15 oz) black beans, drained and rinsed
- 1 can (4 oz) diced green chiles
- 1 tsp ground cumin
- 1 tsp chili powder
- Salt and pepper, to taste
- 8-10 corn tortillas
- 1 cup enchilada sauce
- 1/2 cup shredded vegan cheese (optional)
- Fresh cilantro, for garnish

Preparation:

1. Preheat your oven to 375°F (190°C).
2. In a large skillet, heat the olive oil over medium heat. Add the diced sweet potatoes and cook for 10-12 minutes, until soft.
3. Add the chopped onion and minced garlic to the skillet and cook for an additional 3-5 minutes.
4. Add the drained black beans, diced green chiles, ground cumin, chili powder, salt and pepper to the skillet. Stir to combine and let cook for a few more minutes.
5. Spoon a small amount of the sweet potato and black bean mixture onto each corn tortilla and roll them up tightly. Place them in a 9x13 inch baking dish.
6. Pour the enchilada sauce over the rolled tortillas, making sure they are all covered. If using, sprinkle shredded vegan cheese on top.
7. Bake for 20 minutes, until the tortillas are slightly crispy and the cheese is melted.
8. Serve hot, topped with fresh cilantro. Enjoy!

Spinach and Mushroom Vegan Lasagna

Cook time: 1 hour
Serving: 8 servings
Ingredients:

- 12 lasagna noodles
- 2 tbsp olive oil

- 1 onion, finely chopped
- 3 garlic cloves, minced
- 16 oz white or cremini mushrooms, sliced
- 6 oz baby spinach
- 1 can (14.5 oz) diced tomatoes
- 1 tsp dried oregano
- 1 tsp dried basil
- Salt and pepper, to taste

Tofu "ricotta" ingredients:

- 14 oz firm tofu, drained and crumbled
- 1/4 cup nutritional yeast
- 1 tsp garlic powder
- 1 tsp dried oregano
- 1 tsp dried basil
- 1/4 cup plant-based milk

Preparation:

1. Cook the lasagna noodles according to package instructions. Rinse with cold water and set aside.
2. Preheat your oven to 375°F (190°C).
3. In a large skillet, heat the olive oil over medium heat. Add the chopped onion and minced garlic and cook for 3-5 minutes, until soft.
4. Add the sliced mushrooms to the skillet and cook until soft, about 5-7 minutes.
5. Add the baby spinach to the skillet and cook until wilted, about 2-3 minutes.
6. Add the diced tomatoes, dried oregano, dried basil, salt and pepper to the skillet. Stir to combine and remove from heat.
7. In a separate bowl, mix together the crumbled tofu, nutritional yeast, garlic powder, dried oregano, dried basil, and plant-based milk to create the tofu "ricotta."
8. In a 9x13 inch baking dish, layer 4 lasagna noodles on the bottom. Top with 1/3 of the spinach and mushroom mixture, then a layer of the tofu "ricotta." Repeat these layers two more times, and top with the remaining 4 lasagna noodles.
9. Cover the dish with foil and bake for 30 minutes. Remove the foil and bake for an additional 15 minutes.
10. Let cool for a few minutes before serving. Enjoy!

Creamy Cashew Alfredo with Spinach

Cook time: 25 minutes
Serving: 4 servings
Ingredients:

- 8 oz linguine
- 1 cup raw cashews, soaked in water for at least 2 hours
- 1/2 cup vegetable broth
- 2 garlic cloves, minced
- 1/4 cup nutritional yeast
- 1 tsp dried basil
- 1 tsp dried oregano
- Salt and pepper, to taste
- 2 cups baby spinach
- Fresh parsley, for garnish

Preparation:

1. In a pot of boiling water, cook the linguine according to package instructions. Drain and set aside.
2. In a high-speed blender, combine the drained cashews, vegetable broth, minced garlic, nutritional yeast, dried basil, dried oregano, salt and pepper.
3. Blend until smooth and creamy. If needed, add more vegetable broth for a thinner consistency.
4. In a large pan, heat the cashew alfredo sauce over medium heat. Add the cooked linguine and baby spinach, and cook until the spinach is wilted.
5. Serve hot, garnished with fresh parsley. Enjoy!

Red Curry Vegetables with Coconut Rice

Cook time: 45 minutes
Serving: 4 servings
Ingredients:

- 1 cup white or jasmine rice
- 1 can (15 oz) coconut milk
- 1/4 cup water
- 2 tbsp red curry paste
- 1 onion, thinly sliced
- 1 red bell pepper, thinly sliced
- 1 zucchini, cut into half-moons

- 1 cup chopped broccoli
- 1 can (15 oz) chickpeas, drained and rinsed
- Salt, to taste
- Fresh cilantro, for garnish
- Crushed peanuts, for garnish (optional)

Preparation:

1. In a medium pot, combine the rice, coconut milk, and water. Bring to a boil, then reduce the heat and let simmer for 18-20 minutes, until the rice is cooked and fluffy.
2. In a large skillet or wok, heat 2 tbsp of water (or oil) over medium heat. Add the red curry paste and cook for 1-2 minutes, until fragrant.
3. Add the thinly sliced onion and cook for 3-5 minutes, until softened.
4. Add the sliced red bell pepper, zucchini, chopped broccoli, and drained chickpeas to the skillet. Stir to combine and cook until the vegetables are tender.
5. Season with salt to taste.
6. Serve over the cooked coconut rice, and garnish with fresh cilantro and crushed peanuts (if desired). Enjoy!

Chapter 7: Satisfying Sides

Roasted Garlic Mashed Cauliflower

Cook time: 25 minutes

Serving: 4-6 people

Ingredients:

- 1 head of cauliflower, cut into florets
- 4 cloves of garlic, minced
- 2 tablespoons olive oil
- 1/4 cup plain Greek yogurt
- Salt and pepper to taste

Preparation:

1. Preheat your oven to 400°F (200°C).
2. In a large bowl, toss the cauliflower florets with minced garlic, olive oil, salt, and pepper.
3. Spread the cauliflower mixture on a baking sheet and roast for 20 minutes, until tender.
4. Transfer the roasted cauliflower to a food processor or blender.
5. Add plain Greek yogurt and blend until smooth and creamy.
6. Transfer to a serving dish and top with additional salt and pepper, if desired.
7. Serve warm.

Lemon Herb Quinoa

Cook time: 20 minutes

Serving: 4-6 people

Ingredients:

- 1 cup uncooked quinoa
- 2 cups water
- 1 teaspoon dried thyme
- 1 teaspoon dried oregano
- Zest and juice of 1 lemon
- Salt and pepper to taste

Preparation:

1. Rinse the quinoa in a fine mesh strainer.
2. In a medium pot, bring water to a boil. Add the quinoa and reduce heat to low.
3. Cover and simmer for 15 minutes, until all the water is absorbed.

4. Remove from heat and let it sit for 5 minutes.
5. Fluff the quinoa with a fork and add in thyme, oregano, lemon zest, and lemon juice.
6. Season with salt and pepper to taste.
7. Serve warm.

Sauteed Garlic Spinach

Cook time: 10 minutes
Serving: 4-6 people
Ingredients:

- 1 tablespoon olive oil
- 3 cloves of garlic, minced
- 1 pound baby spinach leaves
- Salt and pepper to taste

Preparation:

1. Heat a large skillet over medium-high heat and add olive oil.
2. Add minced garlic and cook for 1-2 minutes until fragrant.
3. Add spinach leaves and cook until wilted, about 3-5 minutes.
4. Season with salt and pepper to taste.
5. Serve hot.

Balsamic Glazed Brussels Sprouts

Cook time: 25 minutes
Serving: 4-6 people
Ingredients:

- 1 pound Brussels sprouts, halved
- 2 tablespoons balsamic vinegar
- 2 tablespoons olive oil
- 1 tablespoon honey
- Salt and pepper to taste

Preparation:

1. Preheat your oven to 400°F (200°C).
2. In a small bowl, whisk together balsamic vinegar, olive oil, honey, salt, and pepper.
3. In a large bowl, toss Brussels sprouts with the balsamic mixture until evenly coated.
4. Spread the Brussels sprouts on a baking sheet and bake for 20 minutes, stirring halfway through.

5. Serve hot.

Turmeric Roasted Carrots

Cook time: 25 minutes
Serving: 4-6 people
Ingredients:
- 1 pound baby carrots
- 2 tablespoons olive oil
- 1 teaspoon turmeric powder
- Salt and pepper to taste

Preparation:
1. Preheat your oven to 400°F (200°C).
2. In a large bowl, toss carrots with olive oil, turmeric powder, salt, and pepper until evenly coated.
3. Spread the carrots on a baking sheet and bake for 20 minutes, stirring halfway through.
4. Serve hot.

Cucumber and Tomato Salad

Cook time: 10 minutes
Serving: 4-6 people
Ingredients:
- 2 cucumbers, peeled and chopped
- 1 cup cherry tomatoes, halved
- 1/4 cup red onion, chopped
- 2 tablespoons chopped fresh herbs (such as parsley, dill, or basil)
- 2 tablespoons olive oil
- 1 tablespoon lemon juice
- Salt and pepper to taste

Preparation:
1. In a large bowl, combine cucumbers, cherry tomatoes, red onion, and herbs.
2. In a small bowl, whisk together olive oil, lemon juice, salt, and pepper.
3. Pour the dressing over the salad and toss to coat.
4. Serve chilled.

Grilled Asparagus with Lemon

Cook time: 10 minutes

Serving: 4-6 people

Ingredients:

- 1 pound asparagus spears, trimmed
- 2 tablespoons olive oil
- 2 cloves of garlic, minced
- Zest and juice of 1 lemon
- Salt and pepper to taste

Preparation:

1. Preheat your grill to medium-high heat.
2. In a small bowl, mix together olive oil, minced garlic, lemon zest, and lemon juice.
3. Brush the asparagus spears with the lemon mixture.
4. Grill the asparagus for 5-6 minutes, turning occasionally, until tender.
5. Season with salt and pepper to taste.
6. Serve hot.

Roasted Sweet Potatoes with Rosemary

Cook time: 30 minutes

Serving: 4-6 people

Ingredients:

- 2 sweet potatoes, peeled and cut into cubes
- 2 tablespoons olive oil
- 1 teaspoon dried rosemary
- Salt and pepper to taste

Preparation:

1. Preheat your oven to 400°F (200°C).
2. In a large bowl, toss sweet potato cubes with olive oil, rosemary, salt, and pepper.
3. Spread the sweet potatoes on a baking sheet and bake for 25 minutes, stirring halfway through.
4. Serve hot.

Steamed Broccoli with Tahini Drizzle

Cook time: 15 minutes

Serving: 4-6 people

Ingredients:

- 1 pound broccoli florets
- 1/4 cup tahini
- 2 tablespoons lemon juice
- 2 cloves of garlic, minced
- Salt and pepper to taste

Preparation:

1. Fill a large pot with 1-2 inches of water and bring to a boil over medium-high heat.
2. Place a steamer basket inside the pot and add the broccoli florets.
3. Cover and steam for 5-7 minutes, until tender.
4. In a small bowl, whisk together tahini, lemon juice, minced garlic, salt, and pepper.
5. Drizzle the tahini mixture over the steamed broccoli and serve hot.

Brown Rice Pilaf with Mushrooms

Cook time: 30 minutes

Serving: 4-6 people

Ingredients:

- 1 cup uncooked brown rice
- 2 cups vegetable broth
- 1 tablespoon olive oil
- 1 onion, chopped
- 8 ounces mushrooms, sliced
- 2 cloves of garlic, minced
- 1 teaspoon dried thyme
- Salt and pepper to taste

Preparation:

1. In a medium pot, bring vegetable broth to a boil. Add the brown rice and reduce heat to low.
2. Cover and simmer for 20-25 minutes, until all the broth is absorbed and the rice is tender.
3. Heat olive oil in a large skillet over medium-high heat.
4. Add onion, mushrooms, minced garlic, and thyme. Cook until the vegetables are softened, about 5 minutes.

5. Stir in the cooked brown rice and cook for an additional 2-3 minutes.
6. Season with salt and pepper to taste.

Chapter 8: Healing Beverages

Green Smoothie with Kale and Pineapple

Cook time: 5 minutes

Serving: 1-2

Ingredients:

- 1 cup chopped kale
- 1 cup frozen pineapple chunks
- 1 banana
- 1/2 cup almond milk
- 1 tablespoon honey (optional)
- 1/2 cup ice cubes

Preparation:

1. In a blender, combine the chopped kale, frozen pineapple chunks, banana, almond milk, and optional honey.
2. Blend until smooth, adding more almond milk if needed for desired consistency.
3. Add in the ice cubes and blend again until creamy and smooth.
4. Serve immediately and enjoy your nutrient-packed green smoothie.

Golden Milk Turmeric Latte

Cook time: 10 minutes

Serving: 1

Ingredients:

- 1 cup unsweetened almond milk
- 1 teaspoon ground turmeric
- 1/4 teaspoon ground cinnamon
- 1/4 teaspoon ground ginger
- 1 teaspoon honey or maple syrup
- 1/4 teaspoon vanilla extract (optional)

Preparation:

1. In a small saucepan, heat the almond milk over medium heat until warm.

2. Add in the ground turmeric, cinnamon, and ginger, and whisk until well combined.
3. Pour the mixture into a mug and stir in the honey or maple syrup and optional vanilla extract.
4. Enjoy your warm and comforting golden milk turmeric latte.

Fresh Beet and Carrot Juice

Cook time: 5 minutes

Serving: 1-2

Ingredients:

- 1 large beet, peeled and chopped
- 2 carrots, peeled and chopped
- 1 apple, cored and chopped
- 1 inch piece of ginger, peeled
- 1 tablespoon lemon juice

Preparation:

1. In a juicer, add the chopped beet, carrots, apple, and ginger.
2. Juice the ingredients according to your juicer's instructions.
3. Stir in the lemon juice and enjoy the vibrant and healthy beet and carrot juice.

Ginger and Lemon Infused Water

Cook time: 5 minutes

Serving: 1

Ingredients:

- 1 inch piece of ginger, sliced
- 1/2 lemon, sliced
- 4 cups water
- Ice cubes (optional)

Preparation:

1. In a pitcher, add the sliced ginger and lemon.
2. Pour in the water and let it sit for at least 10 minutes to infuse the flavors.
3. Serve over ice cubes, if desired, and enjoy your refreshing and flavorful ginger and lemon infused water.

Antioxidant Berry Blast Smoothie

Cook time: 5 minutes

Serving: 1-2

Ingredients:

- 1 cup mixed berries (such as strawberries, blueberries, and raspberries)
- 1 banana
- 1/2 cup almond milk
- 1 tablespoon chia seeds
- 1 tablespoon honey (optional)
- 1/2 cup ice cubes

Preparation:

1. In a blender, combine the mixed berries, banana, almond milk, chia seeds, and optional honey.
2. Blend until smooth and creamy.
3. Add in the ice cubes and blend again until desired consistency.
4. Pour into a glass and enjoy your delicious and antioxidant-packed smoothie.

Cucumber and Mint Detox Water

Cook time: 5 minutes

Serving: 1

Ingredients:

- 1/2 cucumber, thinly sliced
- 4-5 mint leaves
- 4 cups water
- Ice cubes (optional)

Preparation:

1. In a pitcher, add the thinly sliced cucumber and mint leaves.
2. Pour in the water and let it sit for at least 10 minutes to infuse the flavors.
3. Serve over ice cubes, if desired, and enjoy your refreshing and detoxifying cucumber and mint water.

Matcha Green Tea Smoothie

Cook time: 5 minutes

Serving: 1

Ingredients:

- 1 cup unsweetened almond milk
- 1 banana
- 1/2 teaspoon matcha powder
- 1 tablespoon almond butter
- 1/2 teaspoon honey (optional)
- 1/2 cup ice cubes

Preparation:

1. In a blender, combine the almond milk, banana, matcha powder, almond butter, and optional honey.
2. Blend until smooth and creamy.
3. Add in the ice cubes and blend again until desired consistency.
4. Serve and enjoy your energizing and nutritious matcha green tea smoothie.

Herbal Chamomile Tea

Cook time: 5 minutes
Serving: 1
Ingredients:

- 1 chamomile tea bag
- 1 cup boiling water
- 1 tablespoon honey (optional)
- Lemon wedge (optional)

Preparation:

1. Place the chamomile tea bag in a mug.
2. Pour the boiling water over the tea bag.
3. Let it steep for 3-5 minutes.
4. Remove the tea bag and stir in the optional honey.
5. Squeeze the lemon wedge into the tea for a touch of citrus, if desired.
6. Enjoy your soothing and calming herbal chamomile tea.

Homemade Vegetable Broth

Cook time: 1 hour 30 minutes
Serving: 4 cups
Ingredients:

- 2 tablespoons olive oil
- 1 onion, chopped

- 2 garlic cloves, minced
- 2 celery stalks, chopped
- 2 carrots, peeled and chopped
- 1 parsnip, peeled and chopped
- 1 turnip, peeled and chopped
- 8 cups water
- 1 tablespoon dried thyme
- 1 bay leaf
- Salt and pepper, to taste

Preparation:

1. In a large pot, heat the olive oil over medium heat.
2. Add in the chopped onions and sauté until translucent.
3. Stir in the minced garlic and cook for about 30 seconds.
4. Add in the chopped celery, carrots, parsnip, and turnip.
5. Cook for 5-7 minutes, until the vegetables start to soften.
6. Pour in the water and bring to a boil.
7. Once boiling, reduce the heat to low and add in the dried thyme and bay leaf.
8. Let the broth simmer for 1 hour, stirring occasionally.
9. Remove from heat and let it cool for 5-10 minutes.
10. Strain the broth through a fine mesh sieve and discard the vegetables.
11. Season with salt and pepper to taste.
12. Use immediately or store in the fridge for up to 3 days. Enjoy your homemade vegetable broth in soups, stews, or as a nutrient-dense drink.

Freshly Squeezed Orange Juice

Cook time: 5 minutes

Serving: 1

Ingredients:

- 2-3 oranges
- Ice cubes (optional)
- 4 large oranges
- Water (optional)
- Ice cubes (optional)

Preparation:

1. Begin by washing the oranges thoroughly under cold running water to remove any dirt or residue.
2. Use a sharp knife to cut each orange in half across the middle, creating two equal halves.
3. Take a glass or plastic reamer and insert it into the center of one of the orange halves.
4. Twist and press down firmly on the reamer to extract all the juice from the orange. Do this over a bowl to catch the juice.
5. Repeat the process with all the orange halves until you have extracted all the juice.
6. If you prefer your orange juice without pulp, you can strain the juice through a fine-mesh sieve.
7. If the juice is too tangy for your liking, you can add some water to dilute it to your desired taste.
8. For a refreshing chilled orange juice, add some ice cubes to your serving glasses and pour the juice over it.
9. Give the juice a quick stir and it is now ready to serve.
10. You can store any

Chapter 9: Wholesome Desserts

Chia Seed Pudding with Berries

Cook time: 8 hours (overnight)

Serving: 2

Ingredients:

- 1/4 cup chia seeds
- 1 cup unsweetened almond milk
- 1 tsp vanilla extract
- 1 tbsp maple syrup
- 1 cup mixed berries
- Optional toppings: shredded coconut, sliced almonds

Preparation:

1. In a bowl or jar, mix together chia seeds, almond milk, vanilla extract, and maple syrup. Stir well to combine.
2. Cover and refrigerate for at least 8 hours or overnight.
3. In the morning, give the chia pudding a stir to break up any clumps that may have formed.
4. Serve in bowls or jars and top with mixed berries and optional toppings. Enjoy!

Baked Apples with Cinnamon and Walnuts

Cook time: 40 minutes

Serving: 4

Ingredients:

- 4 apples
- 1 tsp cinnamon
- 1/4 cup chopped walnuts
- 2 tbsp maple syrup
- 1 tbsp melted coconut oil
- 1/4 cup water

Preparation:

1. Preheat oven to 375°F (190°C).
2. Cut off the top of each apple and scoop out the core, leaving a small well in the center.
3. In a small bowl, mix together cinnamon, chopped walnuts, maple syrup and melted coconut oil.

4. Stuff each apple with the cinnamon and walnut mixture.
5. Place apples in a baking dish and pour a 1/4 cup of water into the bottom of the dish.
6. Bake for 30-35 minutes, until apples are soft and tender.
7. Serve warm and enjoy!

Dark Chocolate Avocado Mousse

Cook time: 10 minutes
Serving: 2
Ingredients:
- 1 ripe avocado
- 1/4 cup unsweetened cocoa powder
- 1/4 cup almond milk
- 2 tbsp honey
- 1 tsp vanilla extract
- Pinch of salt
- Optional toppings: chopped dark chocolate, fresh berries

Preparation:
1. In a food processor, blend avocado, cocoa powder, almond milk, honey, vanilla extract, and salt until smooth and creamy.
2. Divide the mousse into serving dishes and chill in the refrigerator for at least 20 minutes.
3. Serve with chopped dark chocolate and fresh berries on top, if desired. Enjoy!

Berry Sorbet

Cook time: 5 hours (includes freezing time)
Serving: 4
Ingredients:
- 3 cups frozen mixed berries
- 1/4 cup honey
- 1/2 cup water
- 1 tsp lemon juice

Preparation:
1. In a blender, blend together frozen berries, honey, water, and lemon juice until smooth.
2. Pour the mixture into a shallow dish and freeze for 1-2 hours.

3. Take the dish out of the freezer and use a fork to break up any ice crystals that have formed.
4. Place back in the freezer and repeat this process every hour for 4-5 hours, until sorbet is firm and smooth.
5. Scoop and serve in bowls. Enjoy!

Almond and Date Energy Bites

Cook time: 20 minutes

Serving: 8-10

Ingredients:

- 1 cup pitted dates
- 1 cup almonds
- 1 tbsp almond butter
- 1 tsp vanilla extract
- 1/4 cup shredded coconut
- 1/4 cup dark chocolate chips

Preparation:

1. In a food processor, blend together dates, almonds, almond butter, and vanilla extract until a sticky dough forms.
2. Roll the mixture into small balls and place on a plate lined with parchment paper.
3. In a small bowl, mix together shredded coconut and dark chocolate chips.
4. Roll the energy bites in the coconut and chocolate mixture until well coated.
5. Place in the refrigerator for at least 10 minutes to firm up before serving. Enjoy!

Coconut and Mango Rice Pudding

Cook time: 45 minutes

Serving: 4

Ingredients:

- 1 cup white rice
- 1 (13.5 oz) can coconut milk
- 1 cup water
- 1/4 cup honey
- 1 tsp vanilla extract

- 1/2 cup chopped mango
- Optional toppings: toasted coconut, sliced almonds

Preparation:

1. In a medium saucepan, combine white rice, coconut milk, water, honey, and vanilla extract.
2. Bring to a boil, then reduce heat to low and let simmer for 15 minutes, stirring occasionally.
3. After 15 minutes, add chopped mango to the rice and continue simmering for an additional 10 minutes, until the rice is fully cooked and the pudding has thickened.
4. Serve in bowls and top with toasted coconut and sliced almonds, if desired. Enjoy!

Greek Yogurt Parfait with Honey and Berries

Cook time: 5 minutes

Serving: 1

Ingredients:

- 1/2 cup plain Greek yogurt
- 1 tbsp honey
- 1/4 cup mixed berries
- 1/4 cup granola

Preparation:

1. In a small bowl, mix together Greek yogurt and honey until well combined.
2. In a glass or jar, layer the yogurt mixture with mixed berries and granola.
3. Repeat the layering process until all ingredients are used up.
4. Top with additional berries and granola, if desired. Enjoy!

Baked Banana Oatmeal Cookies

Cook time: 15 minutes

Serving: 12

Ingredients:

- 2 ripe bananas
- 1/4 cup honey
- 1 tsp vanilla extract
- 1/4 cup coconut oil

- 1 cup rolled oats
- 1/2 cup whole wheat flour
- 1 tsp cinnamon
- 1/2 tsp baking powder
- 1/4 cup dark chocolate chips

Preparation:

1. Preheat oven to 350°F (180°C) and line a baking sheet with parchment paper.
2. In a medium bowl, mash the bananas. Then add honey, vanilla extract, and melted coconut oil. Mix well.
3. In a separate bowl, mix together rolled oats, whole wheat flour, cinnamon, and baking powder.
4. Gradually add the dry ingredients to the wet ingredients and mix until a dough forms.
5. Fold in the dark chocolate chips.
6. Using a spoon, drop the dough onto the prepared baking sheet, leaving some space in between each cookie.
7. Bake for 12-15 minutes, until golden brown. Allow to cool before serving. Enjoy!

Pumpkin Spice Chia Pudding

Cook time: 8 hours (overnight)

Serving: 2

Ingredients:

- 1/4 cup chia seeds
- 1 cup unsweetened almond milk
- 1/4 cup pumpkin puree
- 1 tsp pumpkin pie spice
- 1 tbsp maple syrup
- Optional toppings: chopped pecans, pumpkin seeds

Preparation:

1. In a bowl or jar, mix together chia seeds, almond milk, pumpkin puree, pumpkin pie spice, and maple syrup. Stir well to combine.
2. Cover and refrigerate for at least 8 hours or overnight.
3. In the morning, give the chia pudding a stir to break up any clumps that may have formed.
4. Serve in bowls or jars and top with chopped pecans and pumpkin seeds, if desired. Enjoy!

Lemon Poppy Seed Muffins

Cook time: 25 minutes

Serving: 12

Ingredients:

- 1 1/2 cups all-purpose flour
- 1/2 cup sugar
- 2 tbsp poppy seeds
- 2 tsp baking powder
- 1/4 tsp baking soda
- Pinch of salt
- 1/2 cup unsweetened almond milk
- 1/4 cup melted coconut oil
- 1/4 cup lemon juice
- 2 eggs
- Zest of 1 lemon
- 1 tsp vanilla extract

Preparation:

1. Preheat oven to 350°F (180°C) and line a muffin tin with paper liners.
2. In a large bowl, mix together flour, sugar, poppy seeds, baking powder, baking soda, and salt.
3. In a separate bowl, whisk together almond milk, melted coconut oil, lemon juice, eggs, lemon zest, and vanilla extract.
4. Slowly pour the wet ingredients into the dry ingredients and mix until well combined.
5. Scoop the batter into the prepared muffin tin, filling each cup about 2/3 full.
6. Bake for 20-25 minutes, until a toothpick inserted in the center comes out clean.
7. Allow to cool before serving. Enjoy!

Chapter 10: Meal Plans and Tips

Sample One-Week Meal Plan recipe

Cook time: 30 minutes

Servings: 4

Ingredients:

- 1 pound boneless, skinless chicken breasts, cut into 1-inch pieces
- 1 tablespoon olive oil
- 1/2 onion, chopped
- 2 cloves garlic, minced
- 1 teaspoon lemon zest
- 1/4 cup lemon juice
- 1/2 cup chicken broth
- 1/2 cup uncooked rice
- 1/4 teaspoon salt
- 1/4 teaspoon black pepper

Preparation:

1. Heat the olive oil in a large skillet over medium heat. Add the chicken and cook until browned on all sides.
2. Add the onion, garlic, lemon zest, and lemon juice to the skillet. Cook for 1 minute, or until the onion is softened.
3. Add the chicken broth, rice, salt, and pepper to the skillet. Bring to a boil, then reduce heat to low and simmer for 20 minutes, or until the rice is cooked through.
4. Serve immediately.

Grocery Shopping Guide recipe

Cook time: 30 minutes

Serving: 4 servings

Ingredients:

For the salad:

- 1 head of romaine lettuce, chopped
- 1 cup cherry tomatoes, halved
- 1/2 cucumber, diced
- 1/4 red onion, thinly sliced
- 1/4 cup crumbled feta cheese
- For the dressing:

- 1/4 cup olive oil
- 2 tablespoons red wine vinegar
- 1 teaspoon Dijon mustard
- 1 clove garlic, minced
- Salt and pepper to taste

Preparation:

1. In a large bowl, combine the romaine lettuce, cherry tomatoes, cucumber, red onion, and feta cheese.
2. In a small bowl, whisk together the olive oil, red wine vinegar, Dijon mustard, garlic, salt, and pepper.
3. Pour the dressing over the salad and toss to coat.
4. Serve immediately.

Portion Control Tips

Cook Time: N/A (This recipe is about portion control tips, not a specific dish)

Servings: Variable, depending on your portion control needs

Ingredients:

- Your choice of food or recipe
- A kitchen scale
- Measuring cups and spoons
- Portion control containers (optional)
- Meal planning tools (optional)

Preparation:

1. Choose Your Food: Start with your favorite meal or recipe that you'd like to control the portions of. This can be a homemade dish or a packaged product.
2. Use a Kitchen Scale: Invest in a kitchen scale to accurately measure the weight of your food. Weighing your food is a precise way to control portions.
3. Measuring Cups and Spoons: If you don't have a kitchen scale, use measuring cups and spoons to portion out your food. For example, one cup of cooked rice, half a cup of vegetables, or one tablespoon of salad dressing.
4. Portion Control Containers: Consider using portion control containers, which are designed to help you control your serving sizes. These containers are pre-measured and can be a helpful tool.

5. Divide Your Meals: When preparing a meal, divide it into individual servings based on your portion control goals. For example, if you have a casserole, cut it into equal portions before serving.
6. Plan Ahead: Use meal planning tools, like a weekly meal plan, to ensure you're aware of your portion sizes for the week. This can help you stick to your portion control goals.
7. Be Mindful: Practice mindful eating by paying attention to your hunger and fullness cues. Stop eating when you're satisfied, not overly full.
8. Avoid Eating from the Container: Serve your food on a plate or in a bowl instead of eating directly from a container or bag. This makes it easier to see and control your portion size.
9. Read Nutrition Labels: If you're consuming packaged products, read nutrition labels to understand the recommended serving size and the number of servings per container.
10. Track Your Intake: Consider keeping a food diary or using a smartphone app to track your food intake. This can help you monitor your portion control progress.

Cooking Techniques for Maximum Nutrient Retention recipe

Cook Time: Approximately 20 minutes
Servings: 2
Ingredients:
- 2 cups of mixed vegetables (e.g., broccoli, bell peppers, carrots, snow peas, and mushrooms)
- 1 tablespoon of olive oil
- 2 cloves of garlic, minced
- 1 teaspoon of ginger, minced
- 1 small onion, thinly sliced
- 1 tablespoon of low-sodium soy sauce or tamari
- 1 tablespoon of vegetable broth or water
- Salt and pepper to taste

Preparation:
1. Prep the Vegetables: Wash and chop the mixed vegetables into bite-sized pieces.

2. If using broccoli, blanch it in boiling water for about 2 minutes, then drain and set aside. This helps retain its vibrant green color and nutrients.
3. Sauté Aromatics: Heat the olive oil in a large skillet or wok over medium-high heat.
4. Add the minced garlic and ginger. Sauté for about 30 seconds until fragrant.
5. Add Onions: Add the sliced onions and stir-fry for 2-3 minutes until they become translucent.
6. Stir-Fry Vegetables: Add the prepared mixed vegetables to the skillet. Stir-fry them for about 5-7 minutes, keeping them moving in the pan to prevent overcooking.
7. To help retain nutrients, avoid overcooking the vegetables. They should remain crisp and vibrant.
8. Sauce and Seasoning: In a small bowl, mix the soy sauce (or tamari) and vegetable broth (or water).
9. Pour the sauce over the vegetables and toss to coat evenly.
10. Season with salt and pepper to taste. You can also add a pinch of red pepper flakes if you prefer some heat.
11. Serve: Once the vegetables are cooked to your desired doneness (crisp-tender is ideal for maximum nutrient retention), remove the stir-fry from heat.
12. Serve Hot: Serve your nutrient-rich vegetable stir-fry hot, either as a standalone dish or over cooked brown rice or quinoa for a complete meal.

Mindful Eating Practices

Cook time: 15

Serving: 4

Ingredients:

- A quiet and peaceful place to eat
- A nutritious and balanced meal
- A comfortable chair
- A fork and knife
- Water or tea to drink

Preparation:

1. Set aside time in your day to fully focus on your meal. Turn off all distractions such as TV, phone, and computer.

2. Set up your eating space in a peaceful and clutter-free environment. This could be your dining table or a cozy spot in your home.
3. Begin by taking a few deep breaths and relaxing your body. Allow yourself to fully be in the present moment.
4. Serve yourself a balanced and nutritious meal, taking into consideration portion sizes.
5. Before taking your first bite, take a moment to appreciate the food in front of you. Notice the colors, textures, and smells.
6. Slowly and mindfully chew your food. Pay attention to the flavors and sensations in your mouth.
7. As you eat, try to be present and focus on each bite. Put your fork down between bites and savor the food.
8. Take breaks in between bites to take a few deep breaths and check in with your body. Are you still hungry or satisfied?
9. If thoughts or distractions come up, acknowledge them and gently bring your focus back to your meal.
10. After you have finished eating, take a few deep breaths and notice how your body feels. Give yourself credit for taking the time to nourish your body.
11. Remember to stay hydrated and drink water or tea throughout your meal.
12. Enjoy your meal and try to incorporate these mindful eating practices into your daily routine for a healthier, more mindful relationship with food.

Chicken Stir-Fry

Cook Time: 20 minutes
Serving: 4 servings
Ingredients:

- 1 lb (450g) boneless, skinless chicken breast, sliced
- 2 cups broccoli florets
- 1 red bell pepper, sliced
- 1 small onion, thinly sliced
- 2 cloves garlic, minced
- 1/4 cup soy sauce
- 2 tablespoons sesame oil
- 2 cups cooked rice

Preparation:
1. Heat sesame oil in a large pan over medium-high heat.
2. Add chicken and cook until no longer pink, about 5 minutes.
3. Add garlic, onion, and bell pepper, and sauté for 3-4 minutes.
4. Add broccoli and continue cooking for 2-3 minutes.
5. Pour in soy sauce and cook for an additional 2 minutes.
6. Serve the stir-fry over cooked rice.

Cooking for a Loved One with Cancer

Cook Time: 30 minutes

Servings: 4

Ingredients:
- 1 lb (450g) of carrots, peeled and chopped
- 1 small onion, chopped
- 2-3 cloves of garlic, minced
- 1-inch piece of fresh ginger, peeled and minced
- 4 cups (946ml) of low-sodium vegetable or chicken broth
- 1/2 cup (118ml) of coconut milk (or a dairy-free alternative)
- 2 tablespoons of olive oil
- Salt and pepper to taste
- Fresh parsley or chives for garnish (optional)

Preparation:
1. Heat the olive oil in a large pot over medium heat.
2. Add the chopped onion and cook for about 3-4 minutes until it becomes translucent.
3. Stir in the minced garlic and ginger and sauté for another minute until fragrant.
4. Add the chopped carrots to the pot and stir them with the onion, garlic, and ginger for a few minutes.
5. Pour in the vegetable or chicken broth, and bring the mixture to a boil. Reduce the heat to low, cover the pot, and simmer for about 20-25 minutes or until the carrots are soft and easily pierced with a fork.
6. Using an immersion blender or a regular blender (in batches), puree the soup until it's smooth and creamy. If you're using a regular blender, be careful when blending hot liquids and allow them to cool slightly before blending.

7. Return the pureed soup to the pot, and add the coconut milk. Stir well and heat it over low heat for a few more minutes until it's heated through.
8. Season the soup with salt and pepper to taste. Adjust the seasoning as needed.
9. Serve the creamy carrot ginger soup in bowls, garnished with fresh parsley or chives if desired.

Hydration and Cancer Prevention

Cook Time: 5 minutes
Serving: 4
Ingredients:
- 1 lemon, thinly sliced
- 1/2 cucumber, thinly sliced
- 4 cups of water
- Ice cubes (optional)

Preparation:
1. Wash the lemon and cucumber thoroughly.
2. Slice the lemon and cucumber into thin rounds.
3. In a pitcher, add the lemon and cucumber slices.
4. Pour in 4 cups of water.
5. If you prefer your infused water cold, you can add ice cubes.
6. Allow the water to infuse for at least 30 minutes before serving. For stronger flavors, you can refrigerate the pitcher for a few hours or overnight.

Managing Digestive Symptoms

Cook time: This recipe is all about making lifestyle changes, so there is no actual cooking time.
Serving size: This recipe serves one person, but you can share the tips with others!
Ingredients:
- A healthy diet
- Regular exercise
- Stress management
- Probiotics
- Over-the-counter medications (optional)

Preparation:

1. Eat a healthy diet. This means eating plenty of fruits, vegetables, and whole grains. These foods are high in fiber, which helps to keep your digestive system running smoothly. You should also avoid processed foods, sugary drinks, and excessive amounts of caffeine and alcohol.
2. Exercise regularly. Exercise helps to improve digestion by stimulating muscle contractions in your intestines. Aim for at least 30 minutes of moderate-intensity exercise most days of the week.
3. Manage stress. Stress can exacerbate digestive symptoms, so it's important to find healthy ways to manage it. Some helpful stress-relieving techniques include yoga, meditation, and deep breathing.
4. Take probiotics. Probiotics are live bacteria that are good for your gut health. They can help to improve digestion, reduce inflammation, and boost the immune system. Probiotics are found in some foods, such as yogurt, kefir, and sauerkraut, and they are also available as supplements.
5. Use over-the-counter medications (optional). If your digestive symptoms are severe or persistent, you may want to try over-the-counter medications such as antacids, laxatives, or pain relievers. However, it's important to talk to your doctor before taking any medications, especially if you have any underlying health conditions.

Resources and Support for Cancer Patients

Cook Time: 30 minutes

Serving: 4

Ingredients:

- 1 medium-sized butternut squash, peeled, seeded, and cubed
- 2 large carrots, peeled and chopped
- 1 medium onion, chopped
- 2 cloves garlic, minced
- 1 tablespoon olive oil
- 4 cups low-sodium vegetable broth
- 1 cup canned chickpeas, drained and rinsed
- 1 teaspoon turmeric
- 1/2 teaspoon ground ginger

- 1/2 teaspoon ground cinnamon
- Salt and black pepper to taste
- 1/2 cup Greek yogurt (or a dairy-free alternative for those with dietary restrictions)
- Fresh parsley or cilantro for garnish

Preparation:

1. Heat the olive oil in a large soup pot over medium heat.
2. Add the chopped onion and garlic to the pot and sauté for about 2-3 minutes, or until the onion becomes translucent.
3. Stir in the chopped carrots and cubed butternut squash, and cook for another 5 minutes, stirring occasionally.
4. Add the turmeric, ginger, and cinnamon to the pot, stirring to coat the vegetables with the spices. Cook for an additional minute to enhance the flavors.
5. Pour in the low-sodium vegetable broth, and bring the mixture to a boil. Once it's boiling, reduce the heat to a simmer, cover the pot, and let it cook for about 15-20 minutes or until the vegetables are tender.
6. Using an immersion blender or a regular blender (in batches), carefully puree the soup until it's smooth and creamy. Be cautious when blending hot liquids.
7. Return the pureed soup to the pot and stir in the drained chickpeas. Cook for an additional 5 minutes to heat the chickpeas through.
8. Season the soup with salt and black pepper to taste.
9. Ladle the soup into serving bowls, and top each bowl with a dollop of Greek yogurt (or dairy-free alternative) and a sprinkle of fresh parsley or cilantro.